My Scoliosis Story

One Girl's Journey
From Diagnosis To
Spinal Fusion Surgery

Becky Greulich

Copyright 2019 © by Becky Greulich
All rights reserved.

Except as permitted under the U.S. Copyright Act of 1976, no part of this publication may be reproduced, distributed, or transmitted in any form or by any means, or stored in a database or retrieval system, without the prior permission of the author or publisher. Submit requests to: My Scoliosis Story, 21 Vaughns Gap Road. H141, Nashville, TN 37205

Printed in the United States of America
First Edition: January 2019
Shuffle Street Publishing
Edited by Stuart Englert
Cover photo by Jenna Greulich
Back cover image © CanStockPhoto/Draw05

Library of Congress
Cataloging-in-Publication Data
Greulich, Becky
My Scoliosis Story: One Girl's Journey
From Diagnosis To Spinal Fusion Surgery

Summary: "A teenage girl describes her scoliosis diagnosis and five-year journey from back brace to spinal fusion surgery and recovery."

ISBN: 978-1731559623 (paperback) :
1. Becky Greulich—United States 2. Teenager—United States 3. Indiana—United States. 4. Scoliosis—United States. 5. Back Brace—United States. 6. Spinal Fusion—United States 7. Surgery—United States

Dedicated to everyone with scoliosis.

Acknowledgments

Special thanks to the doctors and nurses who diagnosed, treated and cared for me; to my aunt Angie Rahman and cousin Brett Greulich for driving me to and from doctor appointments; and to all of my family members and friends for their prayers, help and support.

What is Scoliosis?

Scoliosis is a sideways curvature of the spine that most often occurs during the growth spurt just before puberty. Tens of thousands of cases of the disorder are diagnosed in the United States each year. It's more prevalent among girls.

So how do you know if you have scoliosis? Common indicators include uneven shoulders, one that is higher than the other or a shoulder blade that protrudes more than the other. Other indicators are uneven hips and breathing problems due to a reduced area in the chest, which restricts lung expansion. Back pain also is a sign. Scoliosis can be very painful.

The cause of scoliosis is unknown, however, the condition often is present and diagnosed during adolesence. Scoliosis can be present at birth if bones in the spine develop abnormally as a fetus grows inside the mother.

Left untreated, scoliosis can worsen, leading to pain and increased deformity, as well as lung and heart damage.

How Is Scoliosis Treated?

The good news is that scoliosis can be treated. After diagnosis, a person with mild scoliosis may be advised to wear a back brace to prevent the curve from progressing. In more severe cases, in which spinal curvature is 45 to 50 degrees or higher, surgery is required.

Spinal fusion is the most common surgery used to treat scoliosis. The purpose of the procedure is to realign and fuse the curved vertebrae so they heal into a single, solid bone.

During surgery, small pieces of bone are placed into the spaces between the vertebrae so they grow and fuse together. Metal rods are used to hold the spine in place to promote fusion. The rods are attached to the spine by screws, or sometimes hooks and wires.

Depending on the size of the curve, surgery typically lasts four to eight hours. Spinal fusion patients usually are up and walking and ready to go home from the hospital in three to five days.

~A Definite Curve~

Dashing across the yard one sunny summer afternoon, I felt a sharp pain on my left side that I'd never experienced before. I was 10 years old at the time and enjoyed physical activities, such as playing tag and running on my family's farm north of Lamar, Ind., but the pain returned each time I got moving.

As the pain persisted, I noticed that the left side of my rib cage stuck out a little farther than the right. My parents, Michael and Linda Greulich, had no idea what was causing my pain or why my ribs were uneven, so they decided to take me to Dale Family Medicine, a clinic in nearby Dale, Ind., for a physical examination.

During my exam on July 20, 2011, Paula Jochem, the nurse practitioner, told me to bend over. She ran her hand down the length of my backbone and then told me to stand up straight. She checked my chest as well and noticed that my rib cage was not in alignment.

Turning to me, she said: "I believe you have scoliosis."

My mother and I had never heard of scoliosis, so the nurse practitioner explained the medical condition, which she described as an abnormal S- or C-shaped curve in the spine. We were shocked and concerned to hear the news. The nurse practitioner ordered an X-ray and recommended that I see Dr. Randall Loder, a scoliosis specialist in Indianapolis.

In the meantime, we searched the Internet for information and learned that scoliosis treatment requires either wearing a back brace or undergoing fusion surgery, depending on the severity of the spinal curve. The thought of major back surgery filled me with fear and I prayed that I wouldn't need an operation.

The following week, I went to Jasper Memorial Hospital for an X-ray, which revealed an S-shaped curve in my spine. Soon after, my mom made an appointment with Dr. Loder, an orthopedic surgeon at Riley Hospital for Children.

To say the least, I wasn't looking forward to the doctor appointment or the three-hour drive to Indianapolis. My parents and I worried what would happen if I needed surgery. We also were nervous about the upcoming trip to the state capital, the largest city in Indiana with a population of more than 820,000.

Living in the country all of our lives made us wonder how congested and hectic city traffic would be, and if we would get to the doctor's office safely. Because my dad was apprehensive about taking us all the way to Indianapolis, my mom's sister, Angie Rahman, agreed to chauffeur us because she was accustomed to driving in larger cities. That made my dad feel better and lifted a burden off his shoulders.

We remained in suspense as the months, weeks and days passed, and the doctor appointment neared. When Oct. 24 arrived, we left home early in the morning for Angie's house and began the 150-mile trip to Indianapolis. Mile after mile, hour after hour, cornfield after cornfield, my anxiety grew as we got closer to

Indianapolis. We were relieved when we arrived at the doctor's office.

As we walked into Dr. Loder's office, we found a friendly receptionist sitting at the front desk. After Mom signed me in, we sat and waited for what seemed like a long time until my name was called. While I was in the X-ray room, Mom and Angie remained outside the door.

After my X-rays were taken, the nurse led us to another room to wait for the doctor. After a few minutes, Dr. Loder entered the room. He was very friendly as he introduced himself. Soon he sat down in a chair, logged onto a computer and pulled up a black-and-white image of my spine.

We could not believe what we saw. My backbone had a definite curve. The doctor confirmed the nurse practitioner's original diagnosis and told us the curve measured 34 degrees thoracic and 26 degrees lumbar. He recommended treatment to prevent the curvature from getting any worse. He told us I would have to wear a back brace. Upon hearing that, I was not happy at all. I knew right then my life would never be the same.

Dr. Loder said if I didn't wear a brace, the curve in my back would continue to get worse and I may have to end up having surgery. I certainly wanted to avoid back surgery, so my only hope from that point was to do what the doctor said and wear the brace.

After we left Dr. Loder's office, we went directly to Advanced Orthopro a few miles away so I could be measured for a brace. The orthotist measured under my arms, down my sides, around my waist, and the length and width of my chest and back to determine the size of the Boston brace I needed.

Made of high-density plastic and lined with plastic foam, the device would be custom-built to straighten my curved spine. The first Boston brace was developed in the early 1970s by M.E. "Bill" Miller and Dr. John Hall at Boston Children's Hospital in Massachusetts.

Once my back brace was ordered, we began the long drive home, knowing that my scoliosis journey had just begun.

Bracing for the Worst

More than a month passed before my brace was ready. Not knowing what to expect, I was hoping for the best and bracing for the worst.

On Nov. 28, Angie once again drove Mom and me to Indianapolis so we could pick up the brace and visit Dr. Loder. Soon after we arrived at Advanced Orthopro, the orthotist walked into the fitting room and began showing Mom and me how the brace is worn around the torso.

After making sure I was wearing a soft undershirt, he pulled the stiff plastic device open so I could wiggle inside. Then he tightened three Velcro straps on the back of the brace. He explained that the brace must fit snugly so it can do its job of correcting my spinal curve. After it was on, I was very depressed.

Being strapped inside the rigid plastic frame was extremely uncomfortable. I could barely breath and the brace fit so tightly that it pressed hard against my underarms and hips and squeezed my sides and stomach. I wanted to take it off, but I couldn't.

The orthotist said for the first week or so I could wear the brace just a few hours a day. Once I got used to it, however, I had to wear it 23 hours a day. That was dreadful news for me.

At that moment, with my entire upper body being crushed and my irritated skin already turning red, I wanted to cry. I tried to remain strong as I put my T-shirt on and pulled it over the top of the brace, but emotionally and physically I was miserable as we walked out of the office.

With every step I took across the parking lot, the pressure from the brace grew more painful. The worst pain was under my arms and on my sides as I crawled into the back seat of Angie's car and she drove us to Dr. Loder's office.

Once at Riley Hospital for Children, I underwent a series of X-rays to see if the brace was correcting the curve in my spine. Dr. Loder assured us it was. We were all happy to hear that, but that didn't relieve the pain I was experiencing. Dr. Loder reminded me to wear the brace 23 hours a day. He said once I got used to it, the pain would subside.

After we left Dr. Loder's office, we stopped at a Cracker Barrel restaurant for lunch, though I didn't feel like eating. Sitting at the table, I tried to get my mind off the pain by ordering some of my favorite foods: mashed potatoes with gravy, coleslaw and fried chicken. Of course, the brace was pushing on my stomach, which ruined my appetite.

I remember going in the restroom with Mom so she could loosen the straps a little to try to help me feel better, but that didn't improve my attitude or appetite much.

After lunch we headed for home. I wasn't looking forward to the three-hour drive as I tried to get comfortable in the car. Fortunately, I fell asleep midway into the trip. When I woke up, we were at Angie's house.

Before we left for Lamar, Mom decided to let me take the brace off. She thought I'd worn it long enough for the first day. I was relieved to get out of that painful piece of plastic and I enjoyed being free of it for the rest of the evening, though I knew I'd be back in that confining contraption the next morning.

For the first couple of weeks, I faced many challenges adjusting to the brace. The biggest was wearing it to school. Because initially I only wore the brace a few hours a day, Mom would come to Lincoln Trail Elementary before noon so I could remove it in the nurse's station. She took the brace home so I wouldn't have to lug it around all afternoon and carry it on the bus. As the days passed, I slowly got used to wearing the brace and the pain subsided just as Dr. Loder said it would.

Because the brace was under my clothes, no one could see I was wearing it or its multi-colored star design. However, to prevent my pants from sliding down on the slick plastic frame, I had to tuck my shirt inside my blue jeans. At school, some students made fun of me for wearing my clothes that way and others asked why I always tucked my shirt in. I explained to them that I wore a back brace and my pants would fall down if I didn't tuck my shirt in. While most of my schoolmates were considerate and understanding, a few continued to laugh at me for being unfashionable.

Wearing the brace posed other problems as well. Because the brace restricted my movement, I couldn't always do what my classmates could do. For instance, when a teacher told us to sit cross-legged on the floor, I had to sit on one hip with my legs in front of me. Because I couldn't bend during gym class, the teacher made me walk laps around the basketball court while the other students stretched and stared at me. Being different drew attention, and the opportunities for embarrassment increased when I began to wear the brace the entire school day.

I was happy when each school day was over. That's when Mom let me remove the brace so I could take a shower. It felt great to have my skin exposed to the air after suffocating in the brace the whole day. The warm water pouring over me felt even more amazing. Unfortunately, I had to put the brace back on with Mom's help and before long I had to wear it to bed every night.

Sleeping in the brace was difficult, especially at first. I couldn't get comfortable. I had to lie on my back because the sides of the brace protruded too much for me to lie on my side. My mom decided to buy me a soft mattress topper because she thought it might help me sleep better, but that didn't help much. I couldn't feel the softness of the mattress because the brace was so hard. Eventually I managed to get to sleep, but finding a relaxed, cozy position was a nightly routine.

On Dec. 15, 2011, we took a trip to the Advanced Orthopro office in Terre Haute, Ind., to get my brace adjusted. It was my 11th birthday. The reason we went to Terre Haute instead of Indianapolis was because the drive was 30 minutes shorter. When we arrived at our destination, I was taken into a room with Angie and Mom so I could remove my brace. After my brace was off, the orthotist took it into another room to adjust the fit.

While we were waiting, we could hear loud hammering. It sounded as if the orthotist was beating on my brace. Later, he came back in the room and put the brace back on me. As he tightened the Velcro straps, I noticed the brace was much snugger than I was accustomed to. My ribs were squeezed, my stomach compressed and I was in severe pain. The man didn't seem to care. He said the brace had to be tight.

"She has to breathe!" my mom replied.

"Well she is breathing, isn't she?" the orthotist responded.

It was the worst birthday I ever had and the worst experience I encountered during my five-year journey with scoliosis.

Since it was my birthday, Angie and Mom wanted to stop at a Toys R Us store to buy me a gift and hopefully get my mind off my pain. Though I was in agony, I managed to pick out a toy helicopter I thought looked pretty cool before we headed home.

As the next couple of hours dragged on, I stared out the car window, watching the traffic, trying to get my mind off my misery. I cried all the way.

I was happy when we finally got to Angie's house. With Mom's permission, I immediately took off the brace. As soon as it was off, I noticed my skin covered in a red rash from the extreme pressure, which had caused my physical distress. One thing was certain, we wouldn't be returning to Terre Haute.

Embracing the Brace

As 2012 rolled around, important decisions had to be made. While my spinal curvature had stabilized, the daylong road trips were exhausting and time-consuming. Plus, we couldn't expect Angie to drive us to Indianapolis every time my brace needed adjusting or my backbone needed to be X-rayed and evaluated.

Mom called Dale Family Medicine for suggestions. An employee recommended she contact Dr. Brett Weinzapfel at Tri-State Orthopaedics in Evansville, Ind., about an hour's drive from our home. Since we also needed a new orthotist, Tri-State Orthopaedics referred us to Chad Allen at Orthotic and Prosthetic Lab, also in Evansville.

Mom made the appointments and Dad drove us to Evansville in January to see both of them. After being examined by Dr. Weinzapfel, we went to see Chad about my brace. After Chad inspected the brace, he determined it didn't fit me correctly, so he measured me for a new one.

When the new brace arrived, he made sure it fit properly and checked that it applied pressure in the appropriate places.

Adorned with an American flag design that I had selected, the new brace was larger and more comfortable than the one I wore previously. Pleased with our experience, we returned to Evansville for future doctor appointments, X-rays and brace adjustments, which required Chad to trim the plastic frame and periodically add padding to ensure a proper fit as my spinal measurements improved slightly.

Before I knew it, the school year was over and spring was in full swing. Summertime and sweltering weather weren't far behind. My first summer wearing the brace was horrible. As the temperature rose, I perspired and the sweat caused the brace to irritate my skin even more. I got extremely irritable. Without airflow, the skin under my brace couldn't dry when I played or worked outside. I was plagued by heat rash, the brace rubbed sores on my body and when I had an itch, I couldn't scratch the spots beneath the brace.

    I was happy when fall and cooler weather arrived, even though I had to return to school. At the time, I was in sixth grade and had to follow the same routine as the previous semester. I wore the brace the entire school day. After the bus brought me home, I took the brace off for an hour or so. After my evening shower, I put the brace back on before I went to bed.

    I was growing fast, and in a little more than a year I had outgrown my second brace. On March 15, 2013, Chad measured me again and ordered a new one. It took two or three weeks to arrive. I was so happy to be free of the brace during that time. I was more comfortable when I slept at night, and more confident when I went to school. Of course, my freedom came to an end when we picked up the new brace, which was just as confining as the previous two even though it was emblazoned with butterflies. After a few more X-rays and brace adjustments, I graduated from sixth grade and another hot summer was upon me.

During summer break, I attended track camp at Heritage Hills Middle, the school in nearby Lincoln City that I would attend in the fall. I was interested in track because I enjoyed running. Each day, the coach advised attendees to stretch their muscles. Because the brace prevented me from bending, I couldn't do all of the stretches.

During the weeklong camp, I ran sprints, laps around the track and jumped hurdles, but found it difficult to leap while wearing the brace. Also, because the weather was hot, I perspired profusely, which once again made me physically miserable. Had it not been for the brace, I probably would have participated in and enjoyed track.

With summer over, it was time for me to enter seventh grade. I was very nervous on the first day of school. I was a self-conscious adolescent, fearing no one at my new school would like me. I wondered how I could endure another year of wearing loose-fitting shirts and trying to camouflage my brace, hoping students I didn't know wouldn't notice.

Fortunately, some sympathetic staff members aware of my scoliosis and back brace had assigned me an end locker, which I could easily access without being crushed in the rush of students between classes. I also got a doctor's written order that excused me from attending swimming class since I had to wear my brace all day. The first semester of seventh grade went by quickly and was fairly uneventful as I turned 13 near the end of 2013.

When I returned for the second semester in January, my schoolwork got harder. The good news was I had great teachers who helped me with my studies so I could complete seventh grade. The bad news was my spinal curvature started to get worse.

Despite the highs and lows of my life, I was looking forward to summer break because my brother Jason was getting married and I was going be a part of the wedding party. I was so excited during that time. I remember trying on my bridesmaid dress without the brace on. I didn't want to wear the brace during the ceremony or reception, plus the dress was such a perfect fit that I couldn't have worn the brace underneath anyway.

    The wedding was on Sept. 20, 2014. It was a great day for everyone, including me, since I wasn't wearing the brace. I had a wonderful time, posing for family portraits and dancing with my three brothers and family members at Fulda Sportsman Club. However, at the end of the day, my back began to hurt. Mom took me home so I could put on the brace and change clothes. When I did, my back began to feel better. That was the first and only time I actually embraced the brace.

School at Home

When I began eighth grade at Heritage Hills Middle, my schoolwork was even more difficult and my stress level increased. The teachers I had were nice, but they didn't offer me as much help as I'd received the previous school year. My grades began to fall.

In late September, Chad no longer approved of the brace I was wearing because once again I had outgrown it. He measured me for the third time and ordered my fourth brace. In about two weeks the plastic frame, with its faux fur design, arrived. Again, I was depressed and fed up with wearing the annoying and troublesome brace.

Each day when I went to school a group of students made fun of my clothing and me. I began to feel like a loser. I didn't fit in and I had few friends.

At the end of the first semester, my class went on a multiday trip to Washington, D.C. I didn't go. Mom and Dad suggested I stay home because I needed someone to help put on my brace and I didn't want to be a bother to anyone on the trip. I was sad. Not only didn't I get to visit the nation's capital, I had to attend school with a few other students who didn't go on the trip and do homework, all because of my brace.

The rest of the semester couldn't have gotten any worse. Some students continued to criticize my clothing behind my back; I was struggling in algebra and science class; and my overall grades were terrible. In December, I turned 14 and remained a prisoner in my brace.

I began thinking about homeschooling. I was getting tired of the classes I was failing. In fact, some of the subjects I was studying seemed meaningless to me. When in my life would I ever use algebra or the Pythagorean theorem? I also was tired of feeling like a loser because I didn't fit in with the popular crowd. Plus, I couldn't participate in track or run cross-country. What's the point, I thought, of going to school when I could learn just as much and better at home?

With careful consideration and planning, Mom pulled me out of public school during the first full week of the second semester. My homeschooling began Jan. 12, 2015.

I began reading English, science and math textbooks that Mom had ordered online. I enjoyed homeschooling because it was less stressful, and I had more time to master the subjects I was studying. I also learned practical skills, such as how to balance a checkbook, cook a meal and do laundry, which weren't taught in middle school.

On March 23 another X-ray was taken of my spine, which revealed my curve had increased to 35 degrees thoracic and 46 degrees lumbar. My scoliosis had progressed despite my bracing. That same day I saw Chad. Initially he wanted to order another brace for me since I had grown nearly 2 inches taller, but after he consulted with Dr. Weinzapfel, they both agreed I should stop wearing a brace until I saw Dr. John Grimm, an orthopedic surgeon in Evansville.

Now things were getting serious—and scary. While I was worried I would need surgery, I wanted my years of wearing a brace to be over. I also was glad to finally be getting a break from the brace.

On April 16, my parents and I met Dr. Grimm. He said surgery was very likely, but he wanted to see me again in six months to check if my spinal deformity got worse or stayed the same. Those were six long, anxiety-filled months.

In Search of a Surgeon

With the likelihood of surgery in my future, my parents began searching for the most experienced surgeon available. Mom and Dad were not going to let just any doctor operate on me, the baby of the family. During their search, my godmother, Janelle Tyree, informed us that one of her friends knew a couple whose teenage daughter recently had undergone scoliosis surgery.

The girl's name was Kylie and her parents were Trina and Derek Schweikarth of Celestine, Ind. We met the Schweikarths at Wendy's restaurant in nearby Ferdinand in July, a few weeks after Kylie's surgery. They told us about Dr. David Schwartz, the orthopedic surgeon in Fishers, Ind., who had performed Kylie's surgery. They highly recommended him and said he performed several scoliosis surgeries each week. They convinced us he was the best surgeon for the job.

In addition to the information shared by the Schweikarths, my family did its own research on Dr. Schwartz. On the Internet, we discovered that he had graduated from Indiana University with honors in 1983. Five years later he graduated from the medical school at Loyola University in Chicago, followed by a general surgery internship at Loyola and an orthopedic surgery residency at Northwestern University. In 1994, he won the North American Spine Society's Award for Outstanding Research. Impressed by his references and credentials, my parents decided to look no further for a surgeon.

When six months had passed, we returned to Dr. Grimm's office in Evansville. The date was Oct. 20. Unfortunately, an X-ray showed my spinal curvature had progressed, increasing to 48 degrees thoracic and 50 degrees lumbar. After Dr. Grimm told us that corrective surgery was necessary, we informed him that we wanted Dr. Schwartz to perform the operation. Dr. Grimm agreed and offered to call Dr. Schwartz on our behalf to schedule an appointment. At that point, I was nervous about surgery but excited to meet the man who would align my spine and free me from the brace.

We met Dr. Schwartz for the first time on Nov. 24, 2015, after Angie agreed to drive Mom and me to his office in Fishers. He was very friendly and knowledgeable. He agreed that I needed surgery and explained the spinal fusion procedure he would use to correct my curve. He described how he would place a metal rod on each side of my backbone and insert screws in my vertebrae. Next, he would place bone fragments along my spine so that within six months to a year the vertebrae would fuse together. After another doctor's visit and consulting his schedule, we decided that April 18, 2016 would be the date of my surgery.

The rest of the year was distressing and depressing for me, especially after my maternal grandmother, Rose Mae Kline, died on Dec. 11, 2015, four days before I turned 15. I spent my birthday at the funeral home with my beloved grandma, the most kind and caring person I'd ever known.

Mom already had a birthday party planned for me before Grandma died. Mom knew Grandma wouldn't have wanted me to change my plans, so we proceeded with the party. A few friends met me at Homestead Pizza in Ferdinand. I had a great time, though I grieved the loss of Grandma.

I also was troubled by the thought of Dr. Schwartz cutting open my skin, putting 12-inch metal rods in my back and driving titanium screws into my spine. Equally upsetting was the fact that despite wearing that painful, irritating brace for more than three years, I still had to have major back surgery. I was anxious to get the surgery over with and get on with my life.

Fusing My Spine

On April 17, Angie drove Mom and me to Indianapolis. We visited the zoo and ate at Long John Silver's before checking into the Marten House Hotel. The hotel was a block away from Peyton Manning Children's Hospital, where I would have surgery the next day.

Before I went to sleep that night, I wondered how my surgery would turn out, but I was not going to worry. My fate was in God's and Dr. Schwartz' hands. Somehow, I knew everything would be all right. My back would be fixed and I would be as good as new.

Around 5 o'clock the next morning we drove to the hospital. Fortunately, we didn't have far to travel. When we arrived, Mom signed me in at the front desk. We sat and waited a few minutes before a nurse called me into a room so she could draw blood samples from me. Soon I was asked to lie on a hospital bed. A few more nurses came in the room to help me prepare for surgery. They were very kind and knew how to keep me smiling.

As they talked to me, the nurses hooked me up to a monitor so the surgeon would know precisely where to make the incision to avoid damaging the nerves in my back. I felt awkward when they pulled my hair back and rubbed a gel-like substance on my head and back before attaching the wired electrodes.

Before long an anesthesiologist came into the room and talked to Mom and me about the drugs that would put me to sleep. Dr. Schwartz entered next. He assured me everything would be OK and that I was going to be taken good care of. As the nurses rolled me out of the room, I waved goodbye to Mom and Angie.

When we got in the operating room, I wasn't awake for more than a minute or two before the anesthetic took effect and I drifted off too sleep.

I was groggy from the sedation when I awoke. Though my memory is foggy, I recall feeling tired, weak and nauseous from the medication. I didn't have an appetite. All I wanted to do was sleep.

Every few hours a nurse would come into the room and help me roll from my back to my side, or vice versa. I couldn't move on my own.

The next day I woke up early in the morning. I felt like I had enough strength to walk a little. I asked a nurse to help me out of bed. Within a few minutes I was on my feet. Once I was up I was so thankful and relieved. It felt great to move. I walked around the entire hospital floor, with assistance of course. The nurse was impressed how well I was doing.

That same morning, I ate some applesauce and Jell-O for breakfast. I still had a hard time eating, but I felt much better as the day progressed.

Several family members visited and a few friends texted me while I was in the hospital. That made me happy. I missed being at home, on the beautiful farm we lived on and around all the animals, which at the time included three dogs, a cat, two calves and a horse.

I was particularly delighted to see my dad, since he was unable to come the day of my surgery. He visited me on my third day in the hospital, along with my brother Andy and his family.

As we were visiting, Dr. Schwartz walked into the room. He told me that he was pleased with the results of my surgery and that I was doing extremely well. For that reason, he told me I could go home the following day. I was ecstatic to hear that and so were my parents and everyone in my family.

I remained tired and weak when I first got home, and the severe pain along my spine persisted. Fortunately, the muscle relaxers and other medication helped me tolerate the pain.

Two weeks later I returned to Dr. Schwartz' office for a checkup. While my surgery was a success, the doctor gave me some restrictions until my incision healed and my spine fused. I couldn't take a bath or swim for six weeks. I had to shower. I couldn't run for a month, though I was encouraged to walk for exercise. I couldn't take medications such as ibuprofen because it would inhibit bone fusion. I was instructed not to bend, twist, stoop or lift anything more than 10 pounds for at least two months after surgery.

The good news was that within a month my pain was gone. I stopped taking muscle relaxers and I quickly regained my strength. My complete recovery took about three months. I was so grateful to be healthy and back to normal.

During the two years after my surgery, we made four more trips to Indianapolis for X-rays and appointments with Dr. Schwartz, who released me from his care on April 17, 2018.

Nearly three years after surgery, I'm doing great. Other than the 13-inch scar down the middle of my spine, no one can tell I had scoliosis. I haven't had any back pain and I can do almost everything an ordinary 18-year-old can do. I feel truly blessed.

Afterword

Scoliosis is no fun for anyone. For some people, wearing a back brace can prevent the need for future surgery. For others, a brace may not help. It's certainly not the end of the world for those who require an operation.

Fortunately, my surgery was a success. I no longer have to worry about wearing a brace, which for me is a huge relief. It's as if I am a whole new person. My back is straight and I'm free to do most anything, including play basketball with my brother Mark and run across the barnyard without pain. I thank God that I found a wonderful surgeon and caring nurses who helped me through the treatment and recovery process.

The journey is indeed long. For anyone who has been diagnosed with scoliosis, I encourage you to have faith and not let fear get in the way of your treatment or surgery.

Whether you're wearing a brace to avoid surgery or surgery is your only option, being in good hands with the right doctors and surgeons can make all the difference. Have faith in God. That is the number one thing.

www.ingramcontent.com/pod-product-compliance
Lightning Source LLC
Chambersburg PA
CBHW031552210526
45464CB00003B/1275